WINSTON

THE AMAZING DOG

An Upbeat Analogy About Diabetes

Book Two of the You Can Do It! Series

Written by **Eleanor Troutt**

Illustrated by **Michael Swaim**

Winston the Amazing Dog
An Upbeat Analogy About Diabetes

Written by Eleanor troutt
Illustrated by Michael Swaim

This is the second book in the You Can Do It! series for children with diabetes.
The first book in this series, The Little Red Sports Car, is available through
Amazon.com, Kindle and Nook. ISBN: 0-615-13281-2

ISBN-13: 978-1478348498
ISBN-10: 1478348496

Printed in the United States of America

Winston was a circus guard dog. That is--he traveled with a circus and helped guard the animals that performed in the circus. The trainers and other humans depended on him to patrol the grounds at night and warn them of any suspicious activity. And Winston was very proud to hold such a responsible position. Life was good!

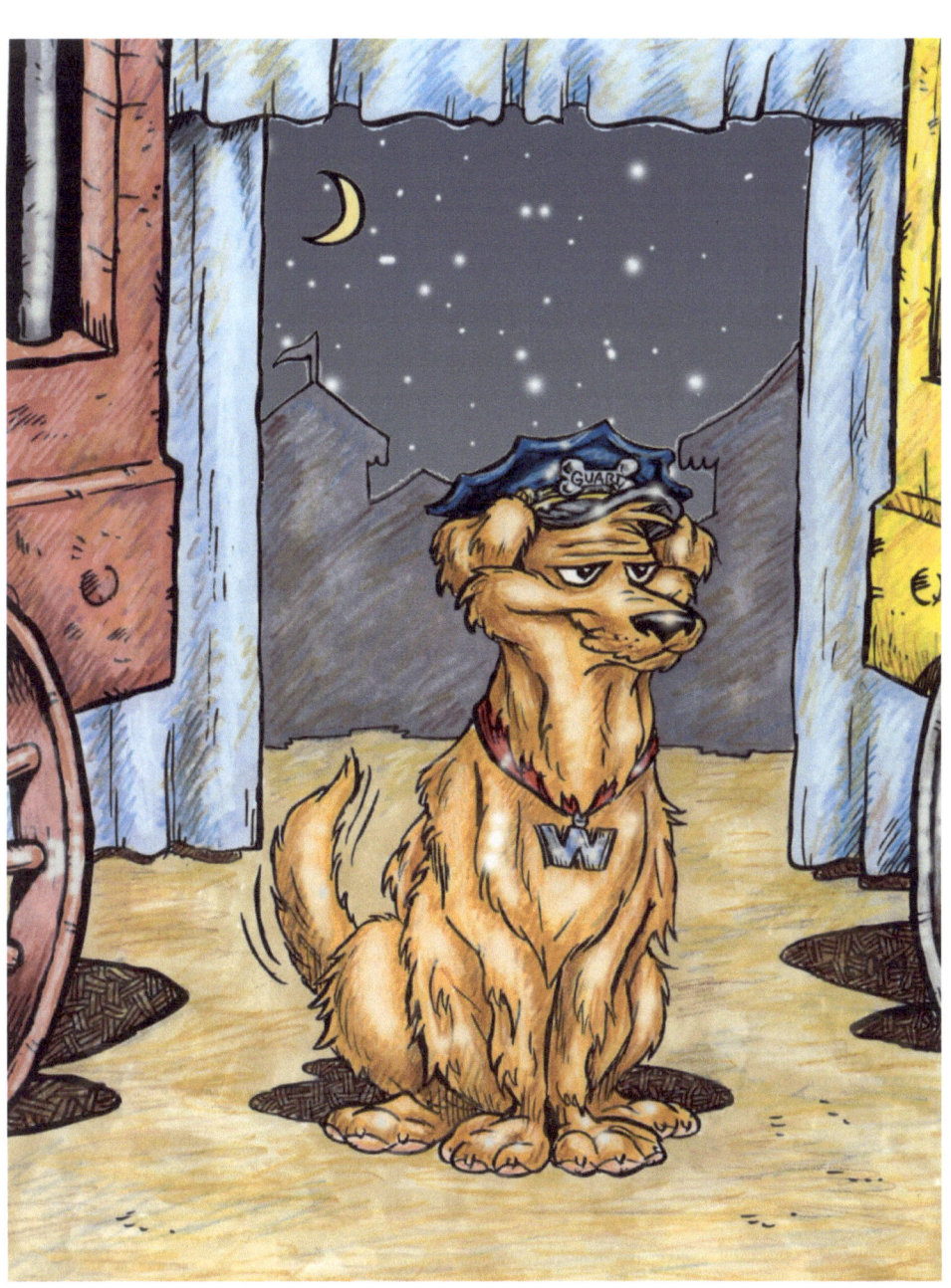

During the day, when he wasn't sleeping, Winston loved to watch the beautiful horses and was intrigued by the way they performed flawlessly to the great delight of the crowds.
He especially liked to watch the stunt riders. How they could swing on and off the horses and balance on them at full gallop completely captivated him!

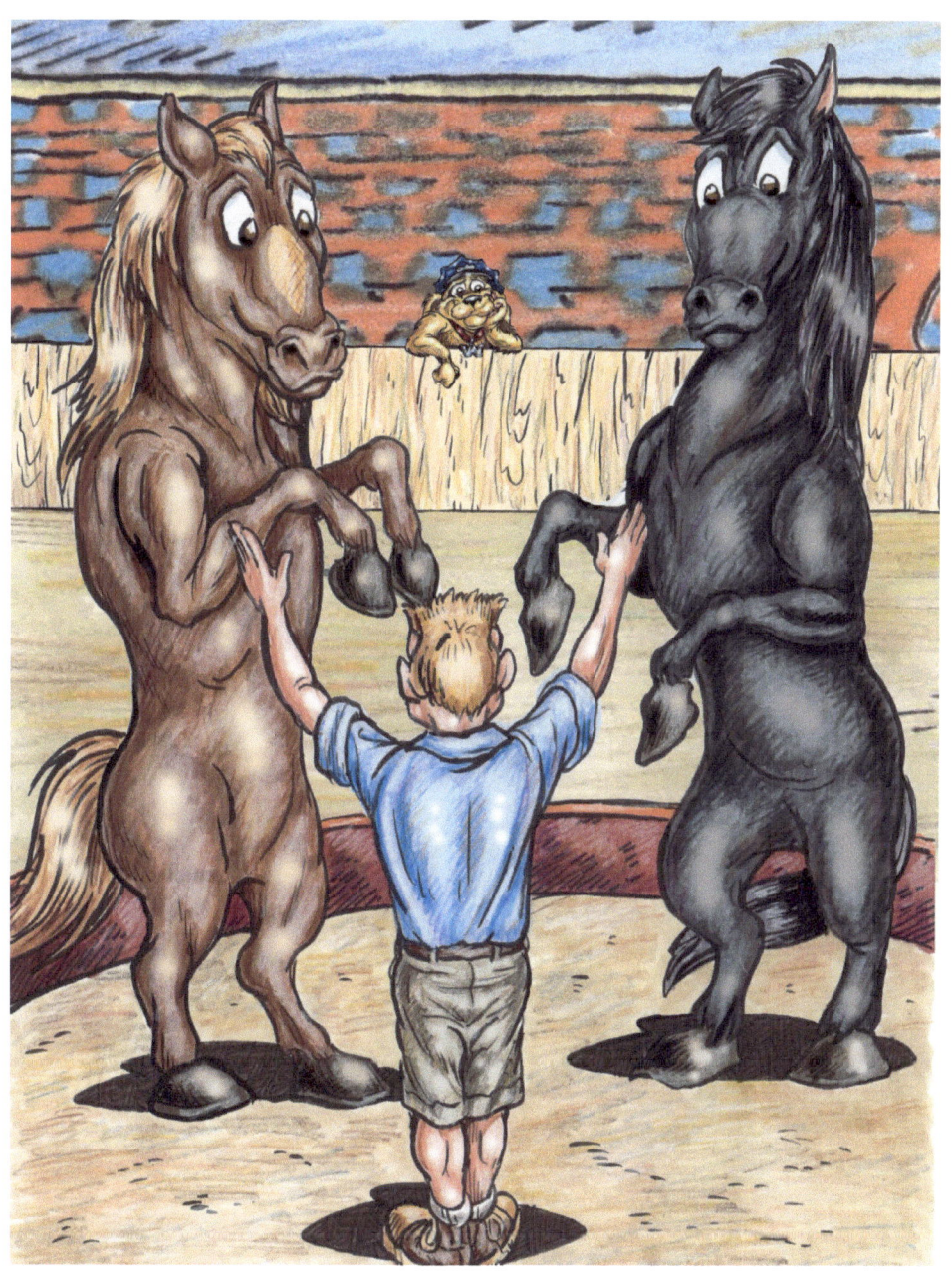

One day he stopped to watch as Max, the trainer, was teaching the horses and the humans a new routine. One of the humans, a beautiful blond lady called Sandy, was learning to balance on the back of a beautiful black pony called Lightning while he galloped around the central ring. It wasn't an easy trick and Sandy was having trouble staying on Lightning's back.

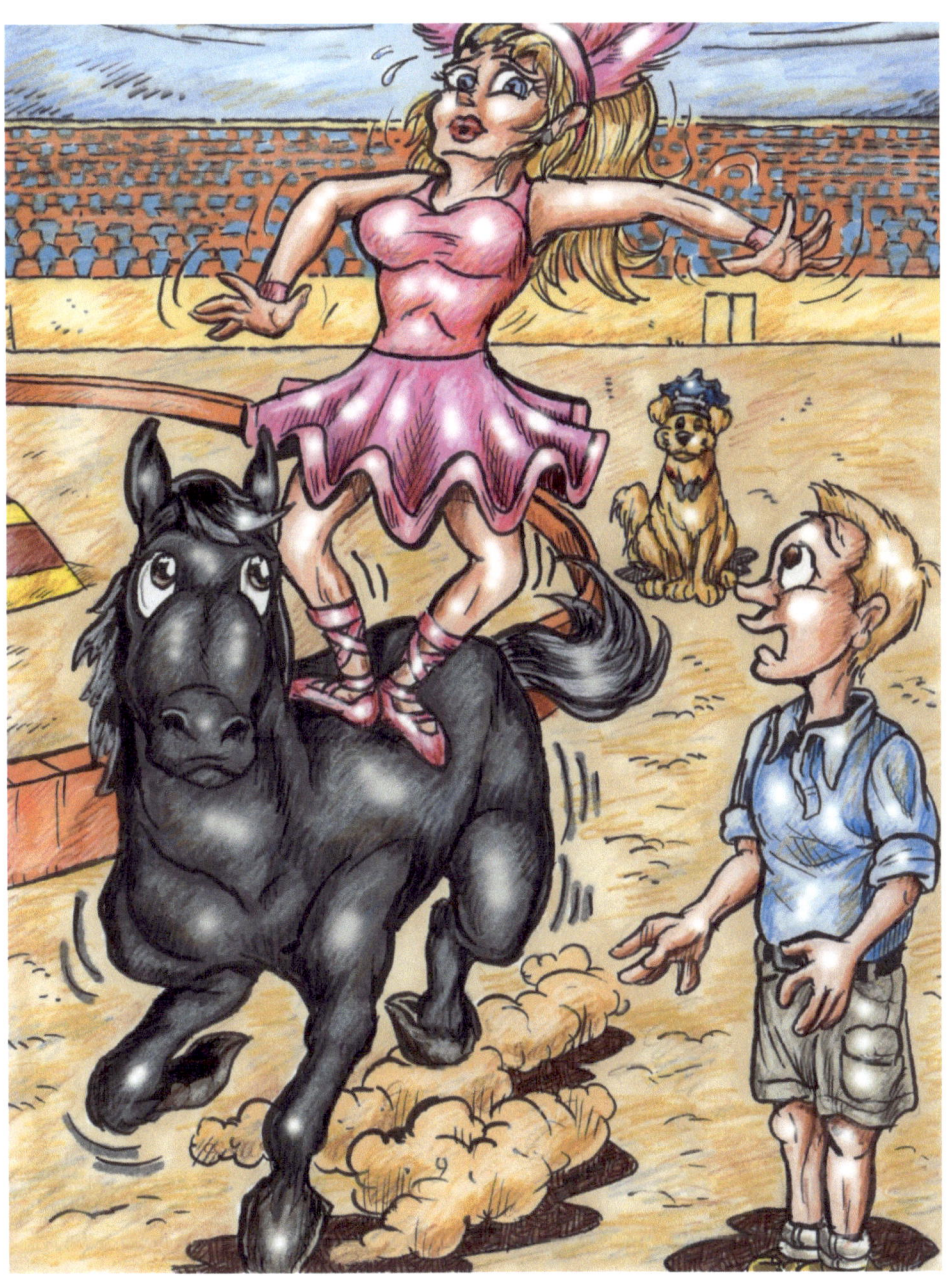

Winston watched for awhile
and decided that it didn't look
THAT difficult! Maybe HE could
do it! He watched for his chance
and when Sandy took a break,
he jumped up on Lightning's
back and quietly barked, "Go".
At first Lightning didn't know
what to do.......

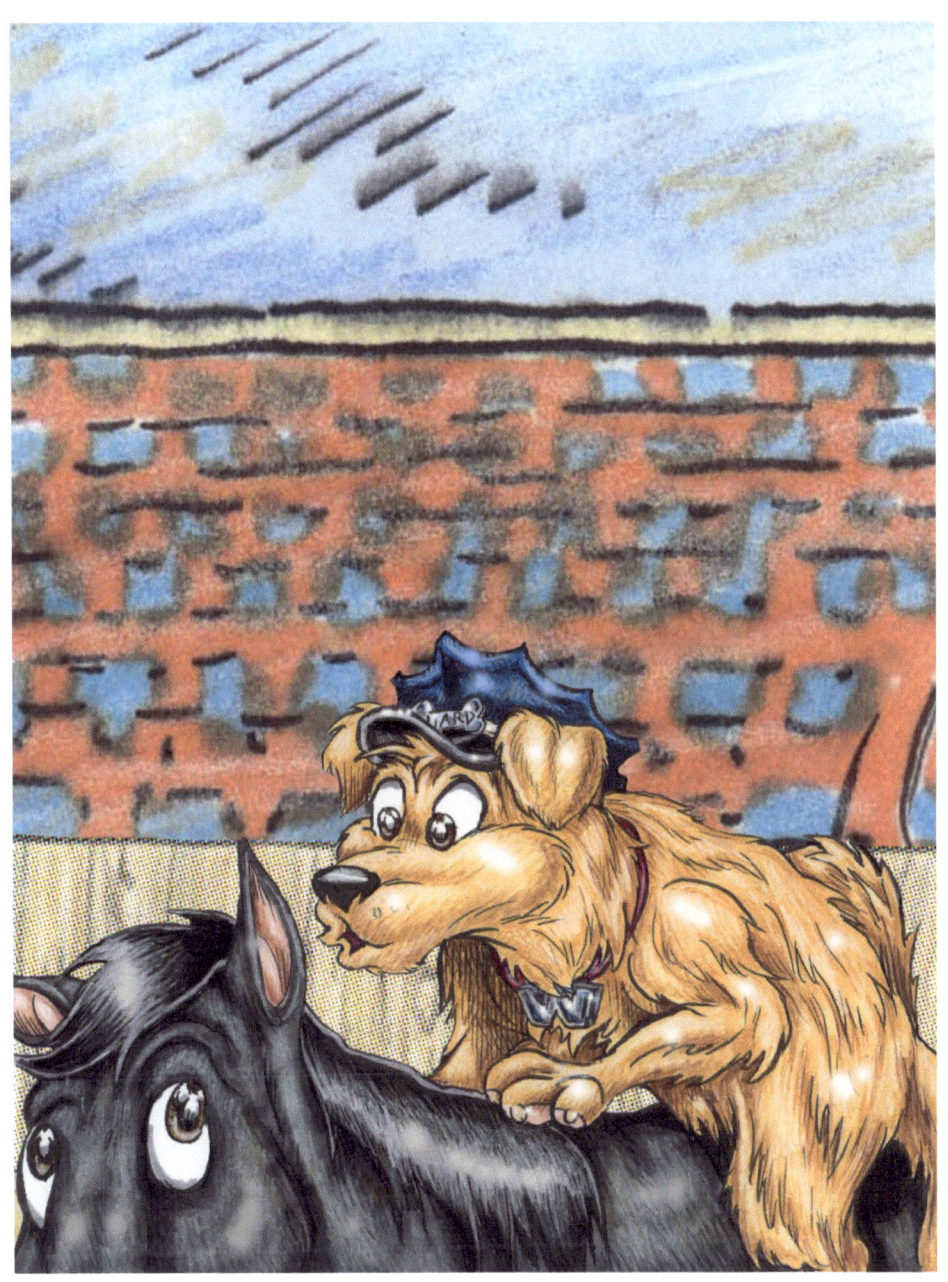

Everyone watched, fascinated at the sight of a dog balancing on the back of a galloping pony. Somehow Winston not only DIDN'T fall off, but he actually put on a very fine balancing act. This wasn't missed on Max. It gave him an idea----why not make Winston part of the act!

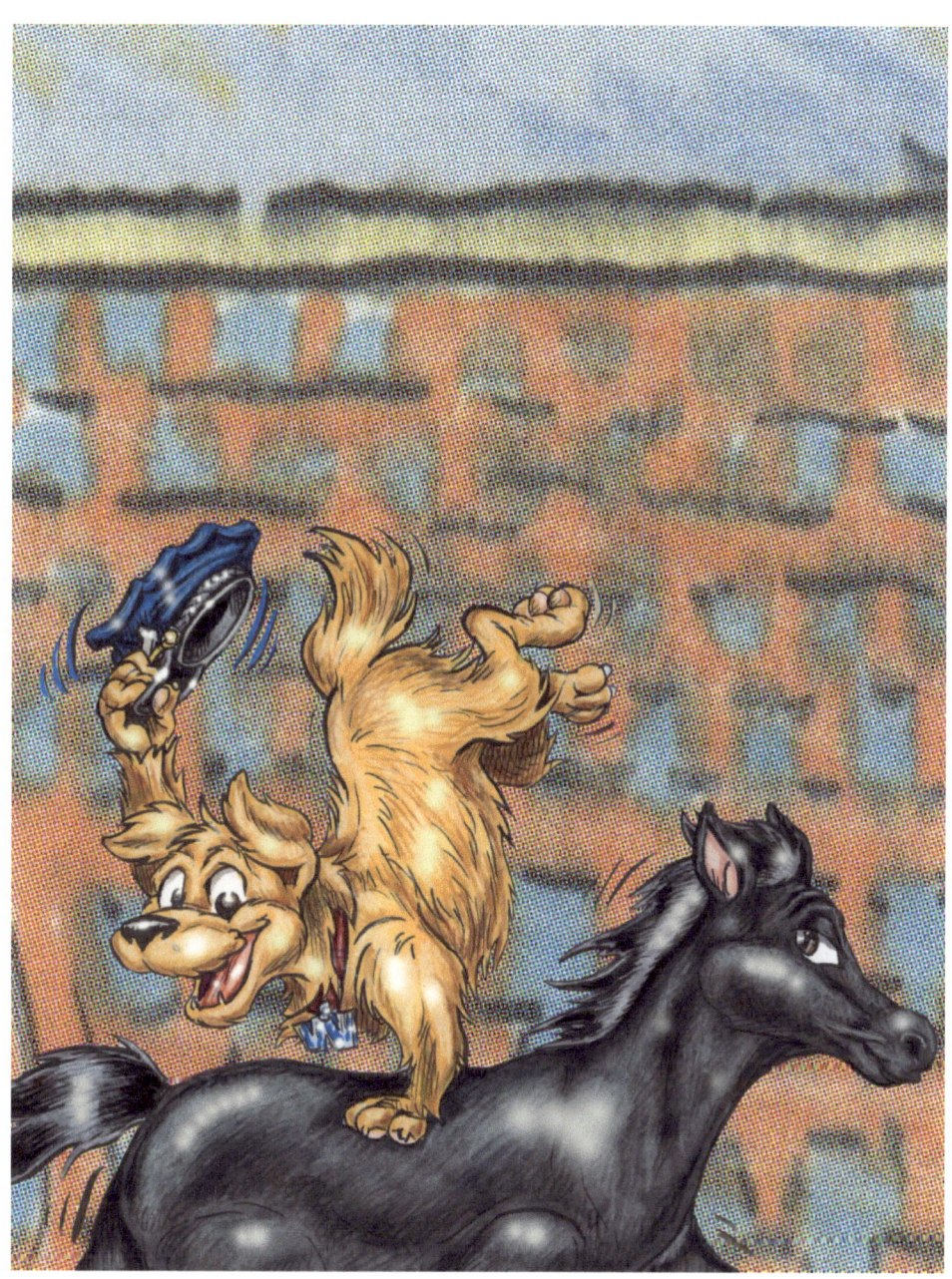

Another dog was brought in
to do guard duty, and in the days
that followed, Max and Winston
worked to perfect the act,
and Winston was outfitted with
a very fine costume for his new
role as a circus performer!

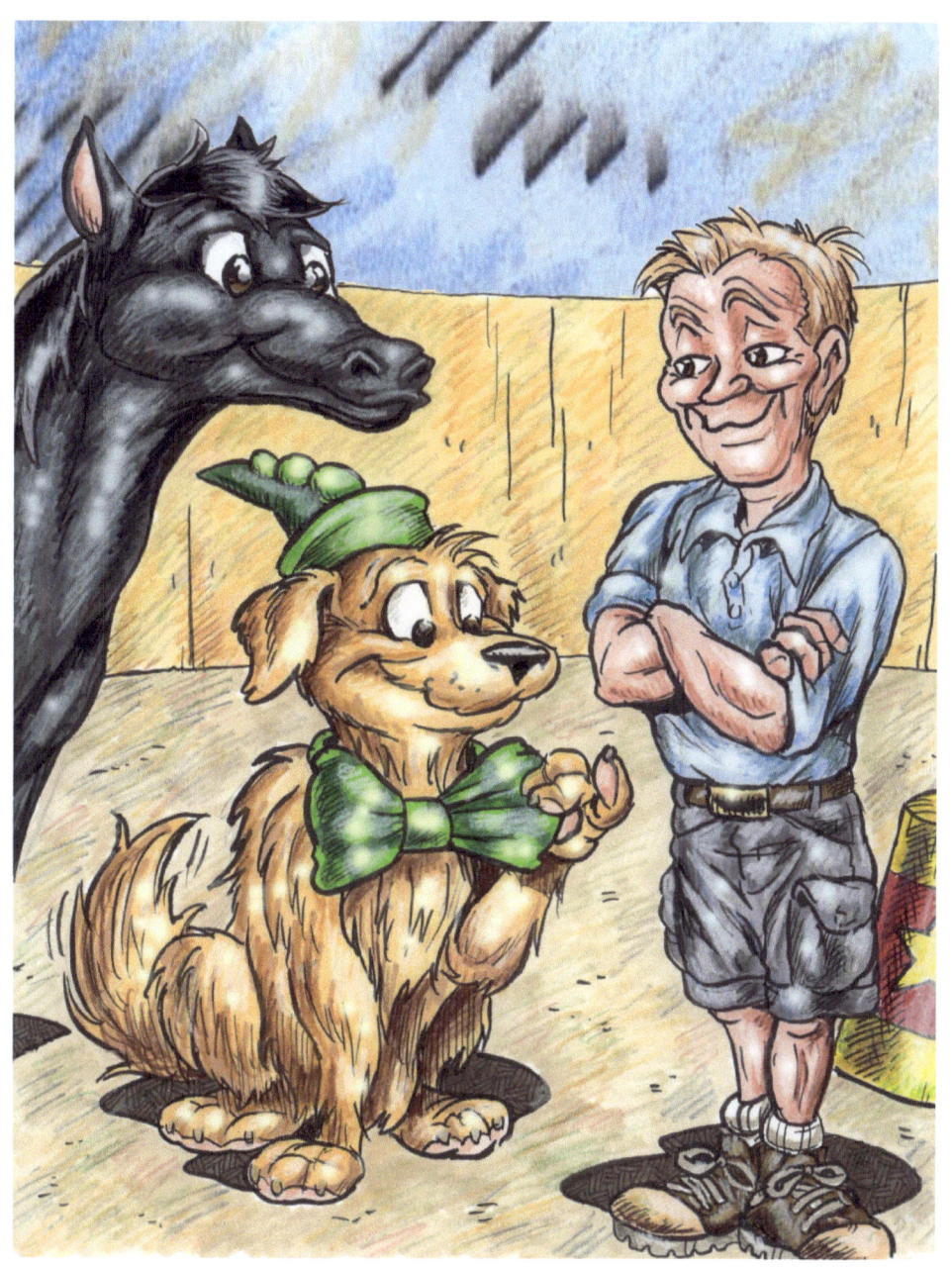

However, something was about to happen which would change Winston's life forever. He hadn't been feeling well for some time, and it was becoming harder and harder for him to perform......

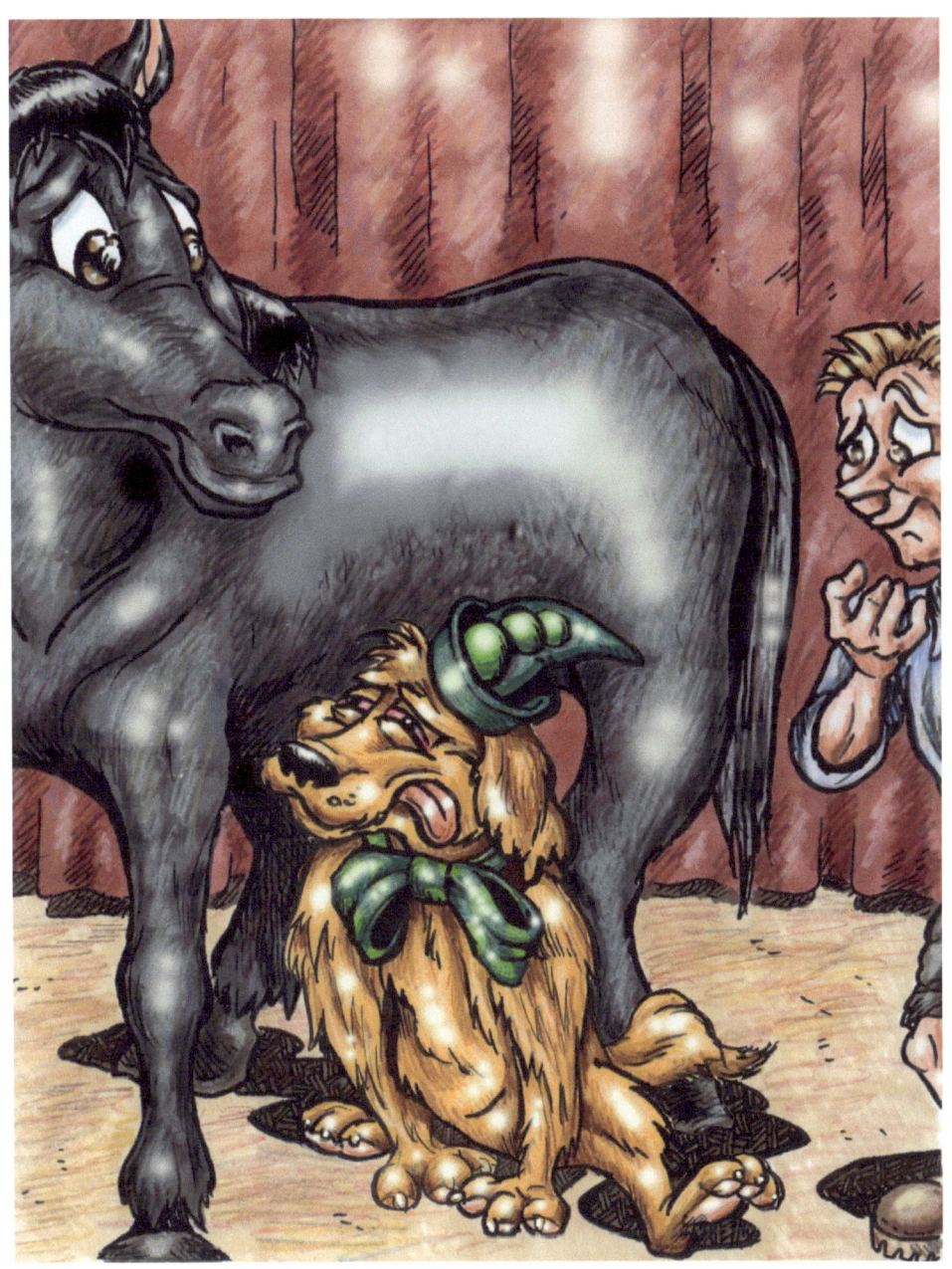

Max was concerned and took Winston to see the veterinarian who often treated animals traveling with the circus. The doctor ran some tests and sadly reached the conclusion that Winston had come down with type 1 diabetes.

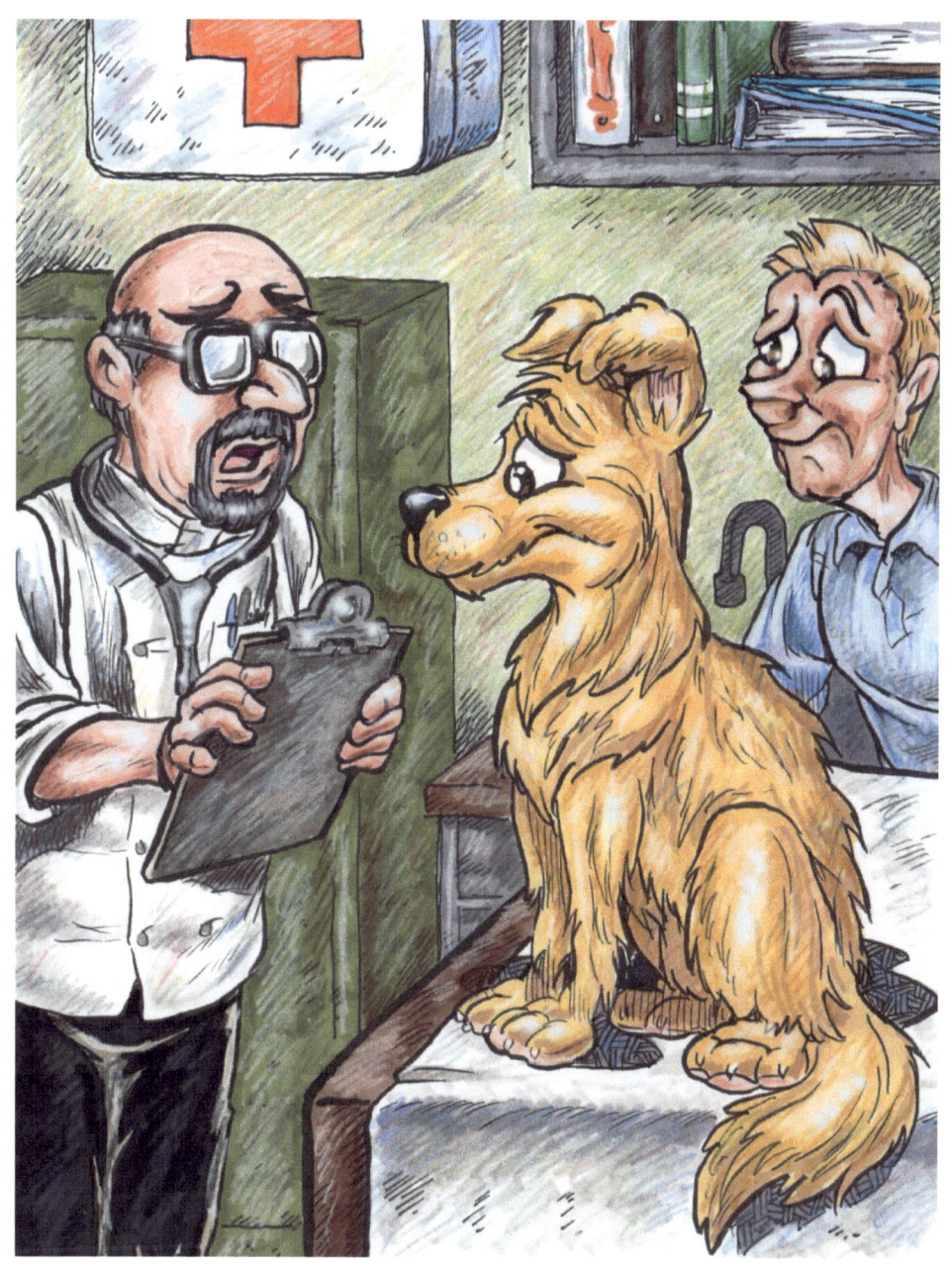

Winston was devastated! He was sure that his circus career was over!

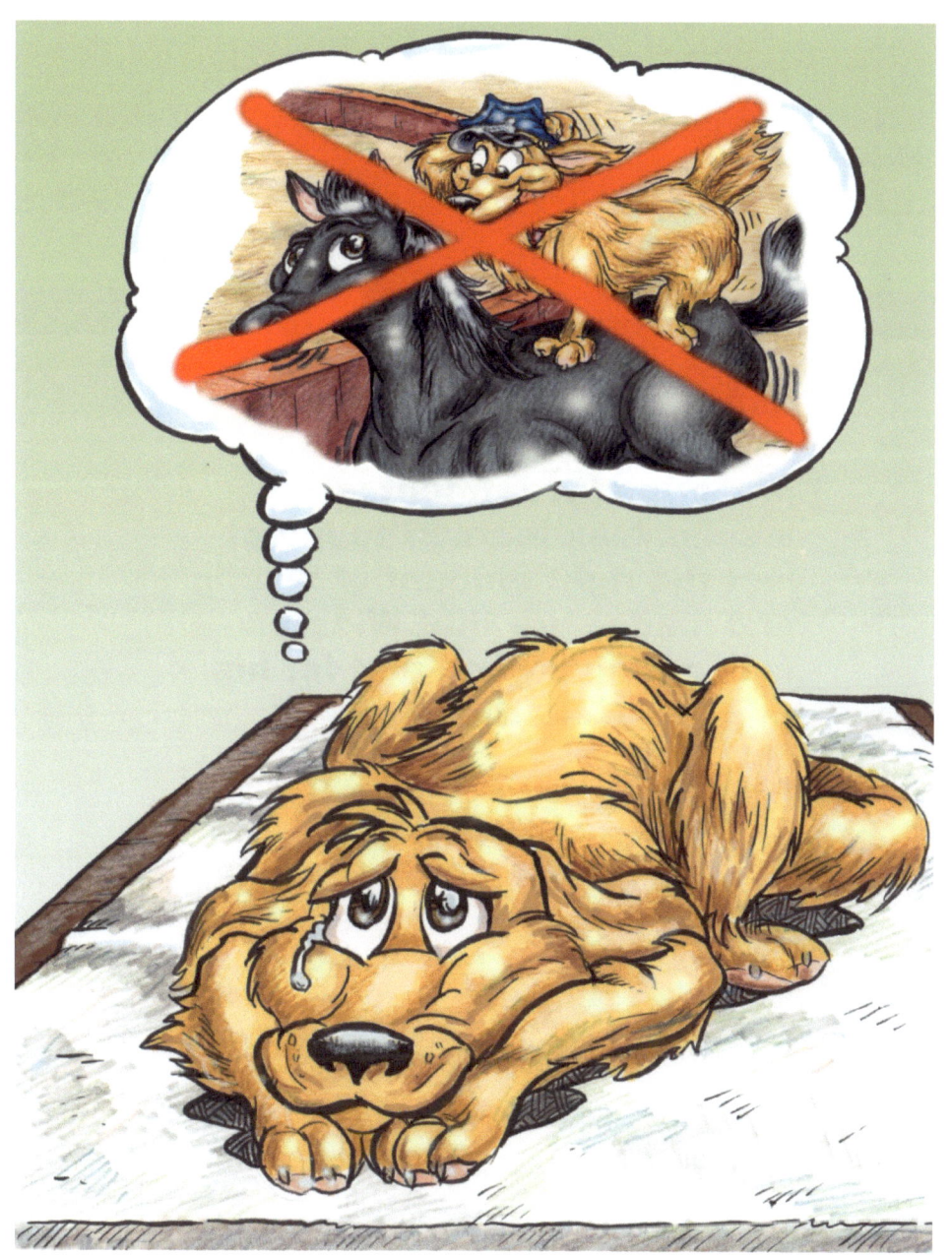

However, the doctor didn't think so. He gave Max some special instructions and prescribed treatment with insulin. Max learned to inject just the right amount of insulin and made sure that Winston was eating a good diet for his condition.

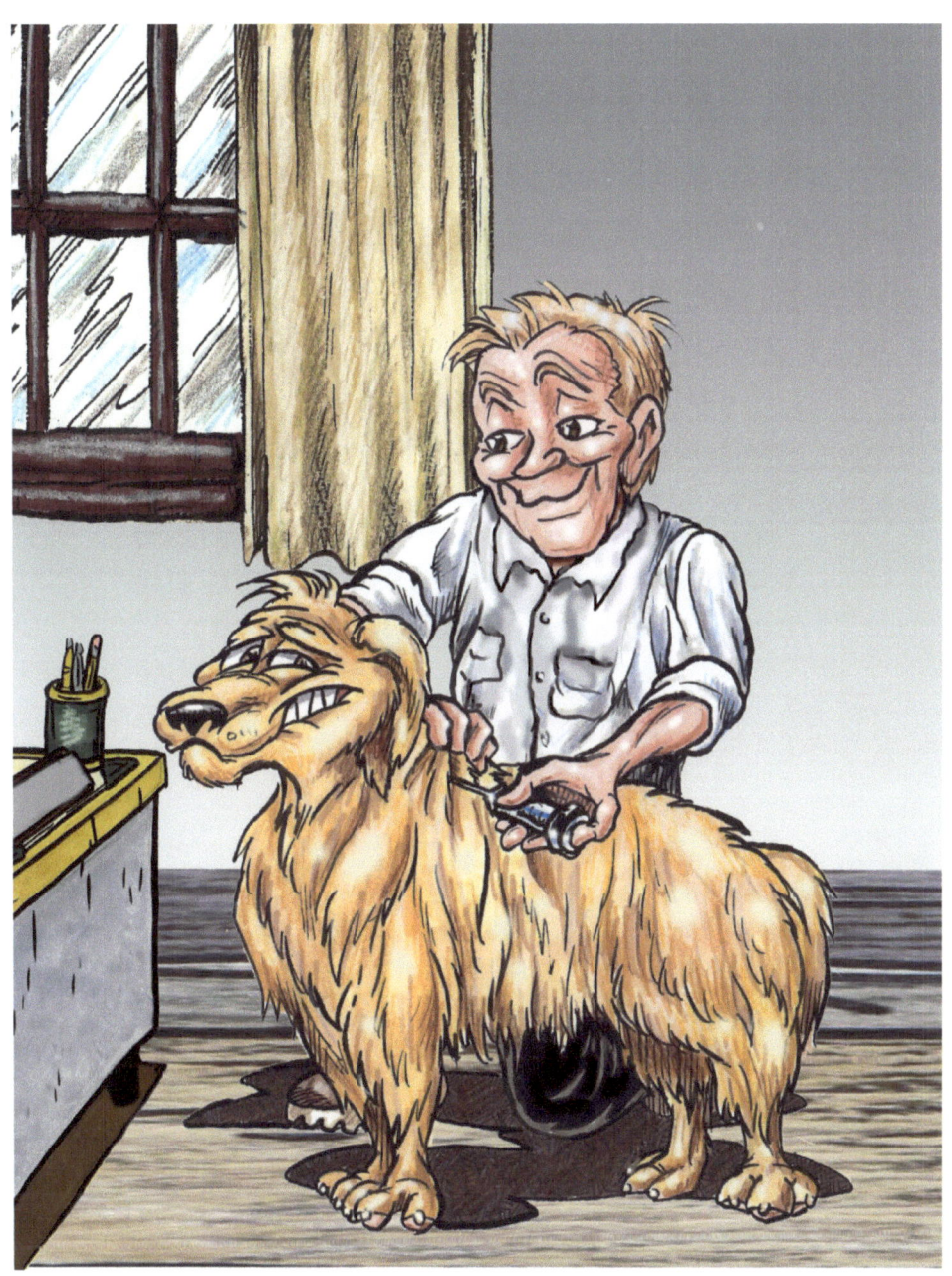

Winston didn't like the shots that Max had to give him every day, but he felt so much better that he put up with it. And before long, he was able to return to the circus and perform his act as usual.

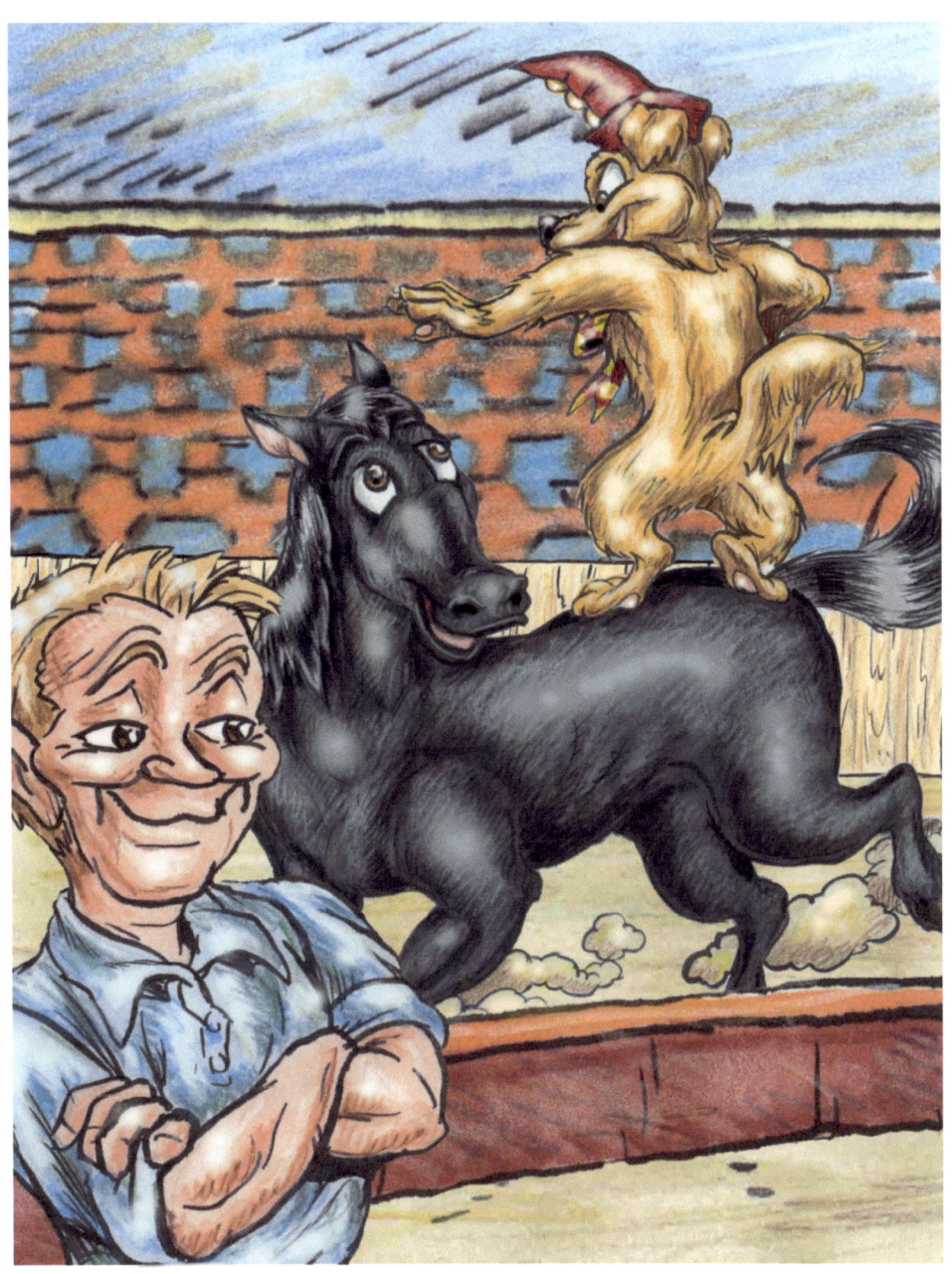

One day a beautiful white pony called Snowflake was brought into the ring and trained to perform the same stunt as Lightning. Then Sandy was asked to perform the very difficult task of balancing on both horses at the same time as they galloped around the central show ring. Winston watched with interest. If SHE could do it, then why couldn't HE?

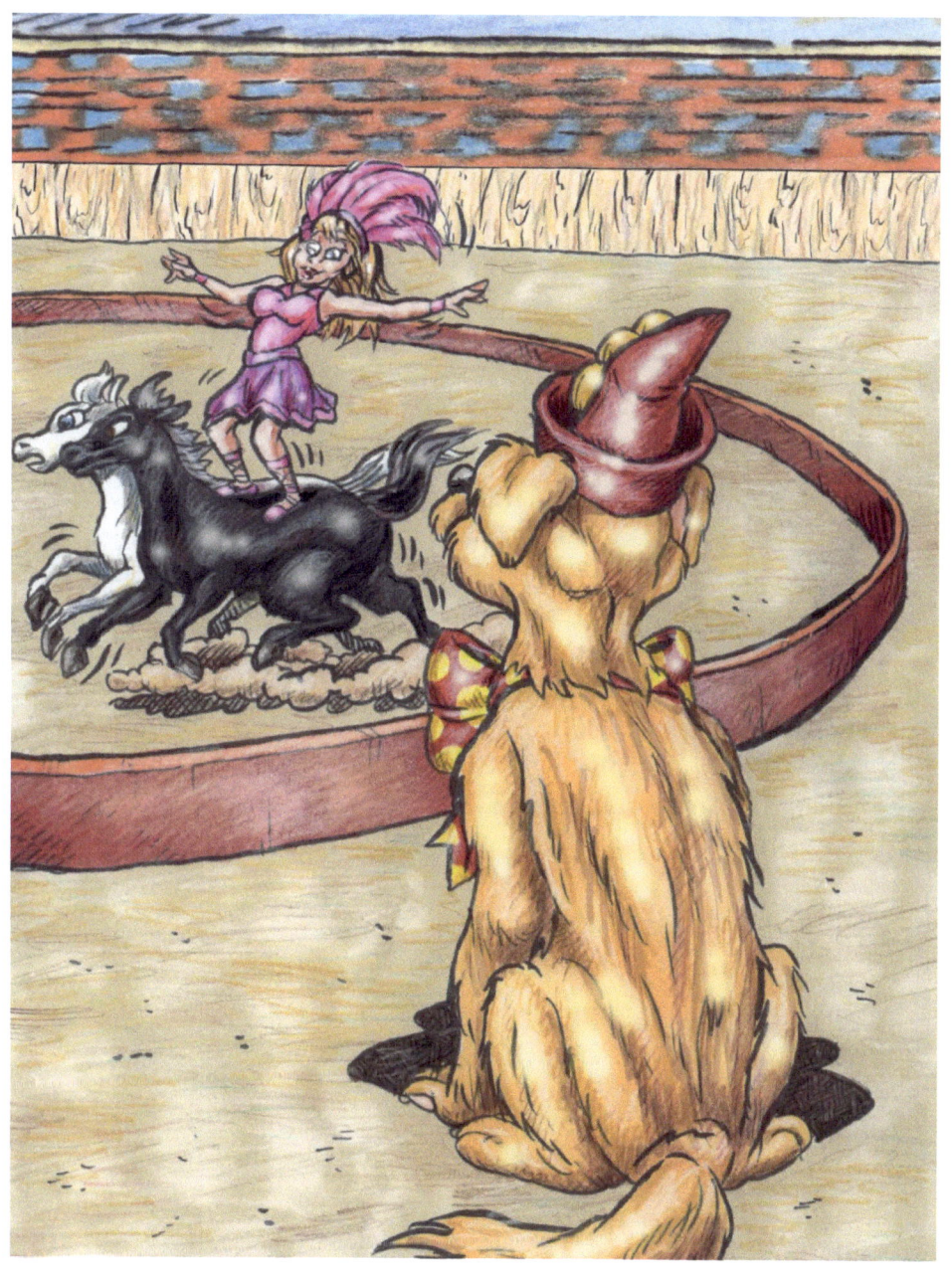

So again, he waited for his chance, and when Sandy and Max weren't looking, Winston hopped up on the back of Lightning and barked for Snowflake to come alongside. Then he quietly barked, "Go".

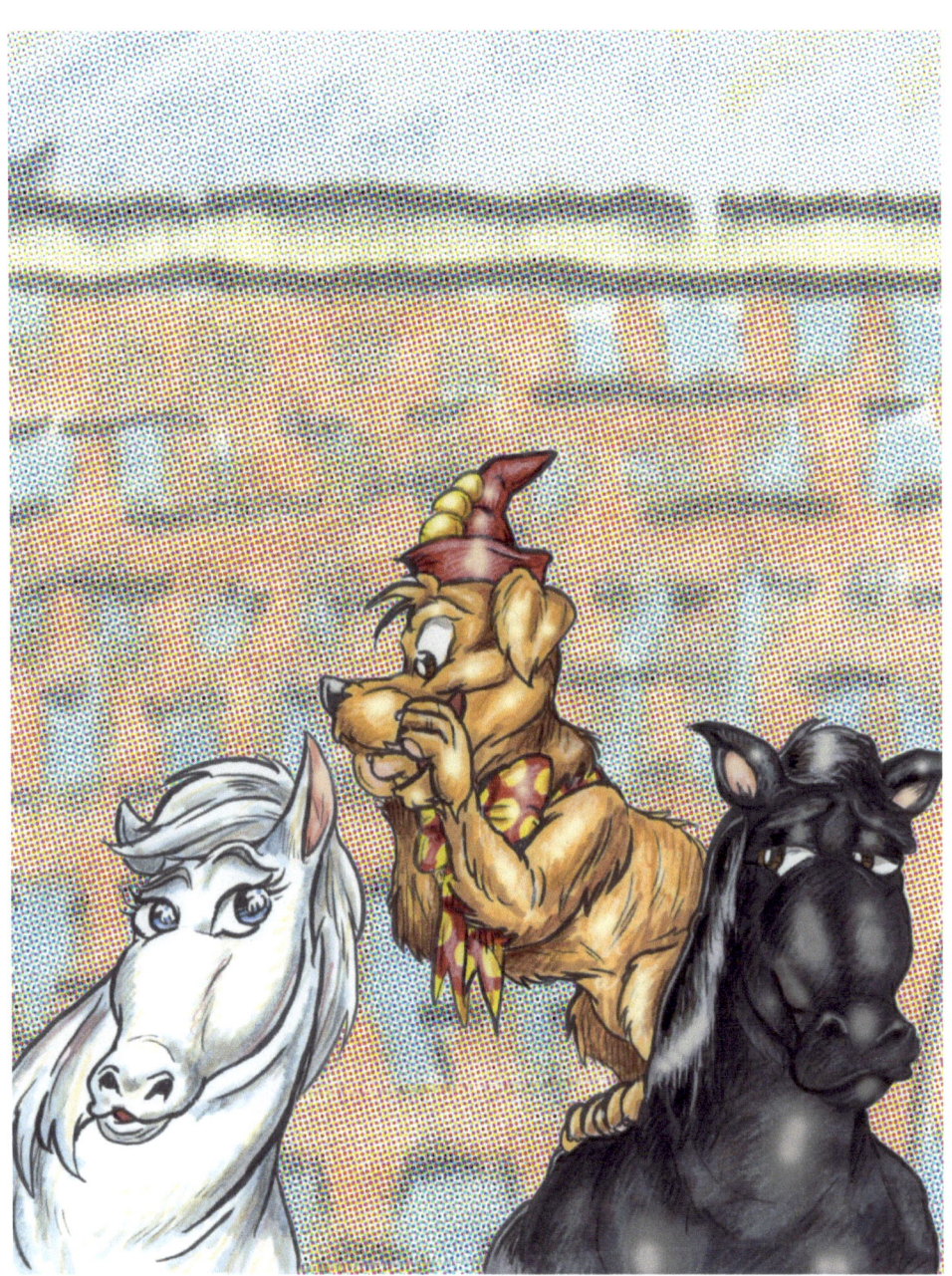

Both horses took off at a gallop with Winston skillfully balancing on BOTH horses. Everyone gasped in amazement! They had never seen such a thing! Of course, this act was also added to the program.....

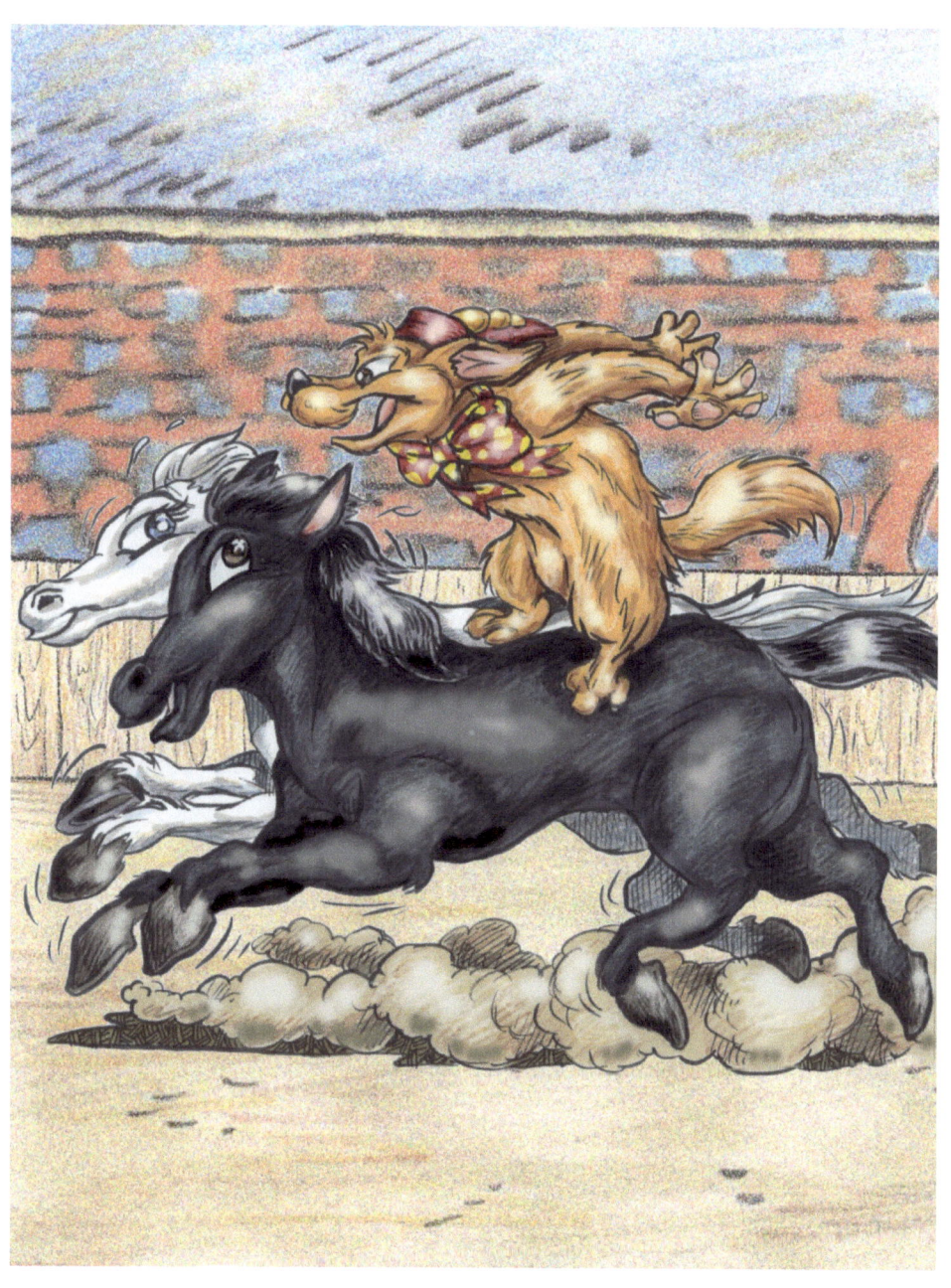

And Winston became a celebrity! They advertised him as "Winston, the Amazing Dog", and families came from all over just to see this unique circus act.

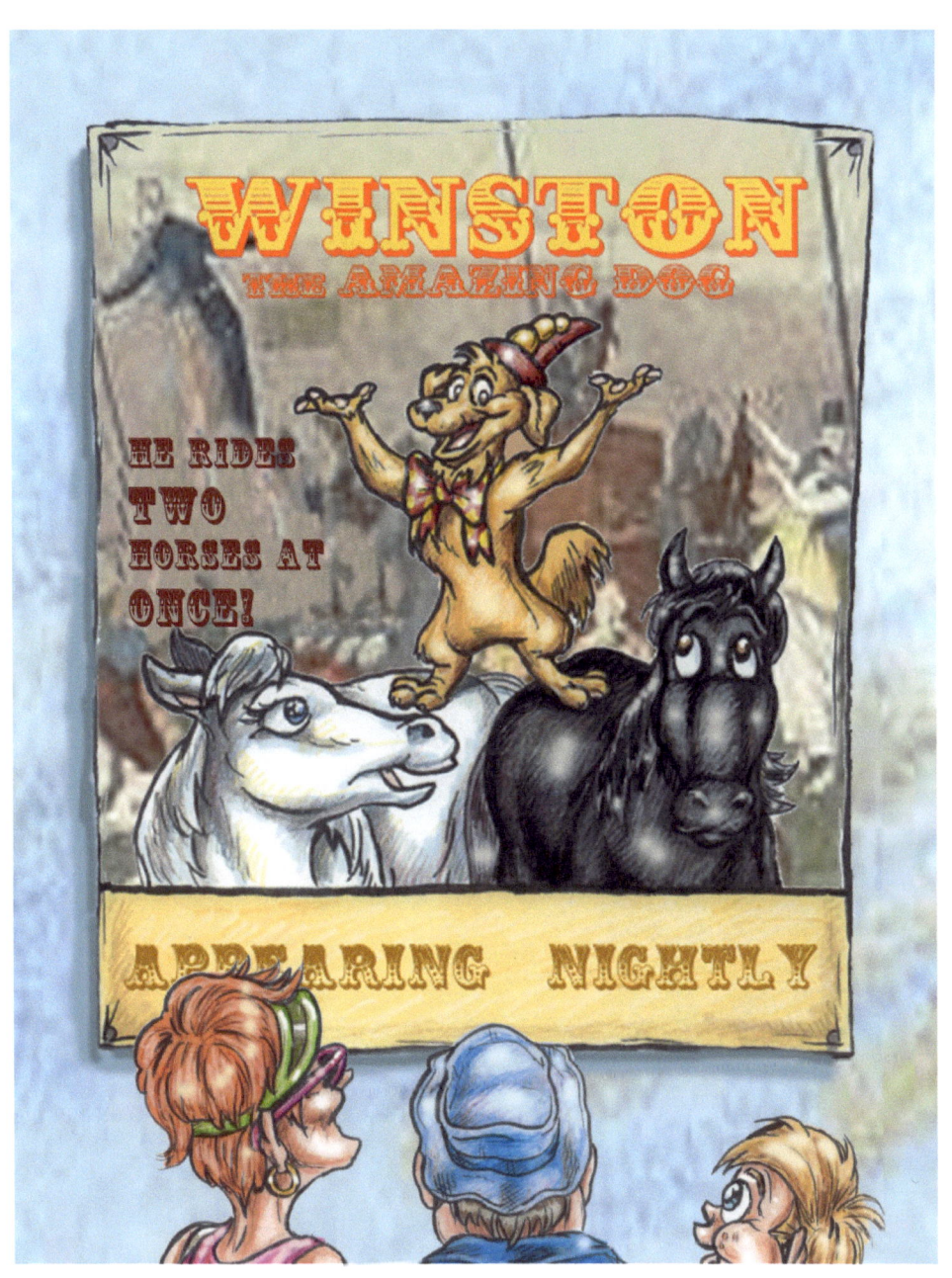

As Winston lay in his kennel one night, he was thinking about his life and how he had been able to continue to do the things he wanted to do in SPITE of having diabetes. After all, he was a famous circus performer, and even after he had been diagnosed with diabetes, he had been able to make the stunt he performed in the circus even MORE amazing.

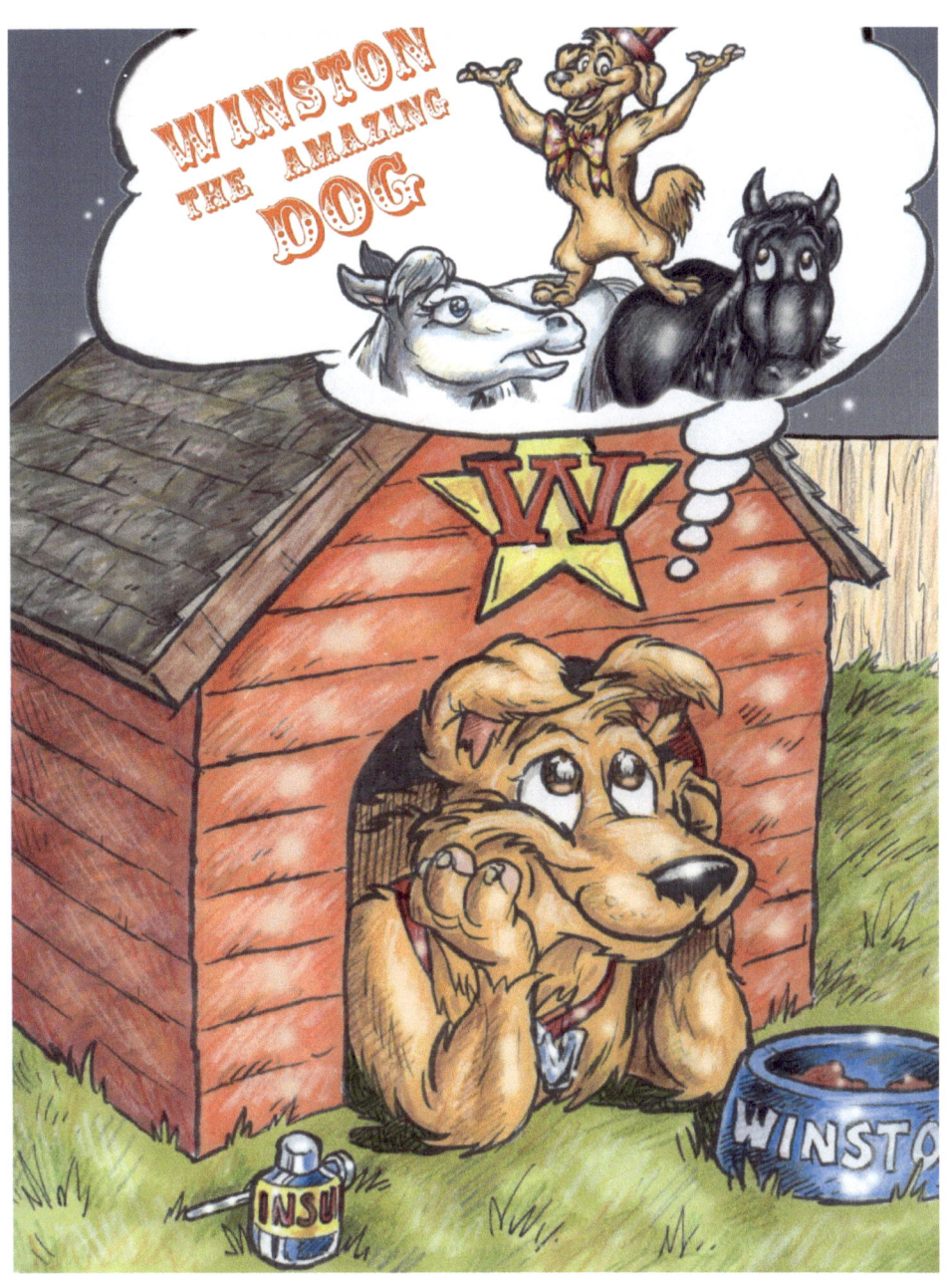

As he thought about this, he realized that performing his balancing act on the backs of two galloping ponies and controlling his diabetes were actually very similar. In both cases he was performing a balancing act.....but in the case of diabetes, he had to balance his life between low blood sugar on the one hand and high blood sugar on the other.

Blood Sugar Levels Chart

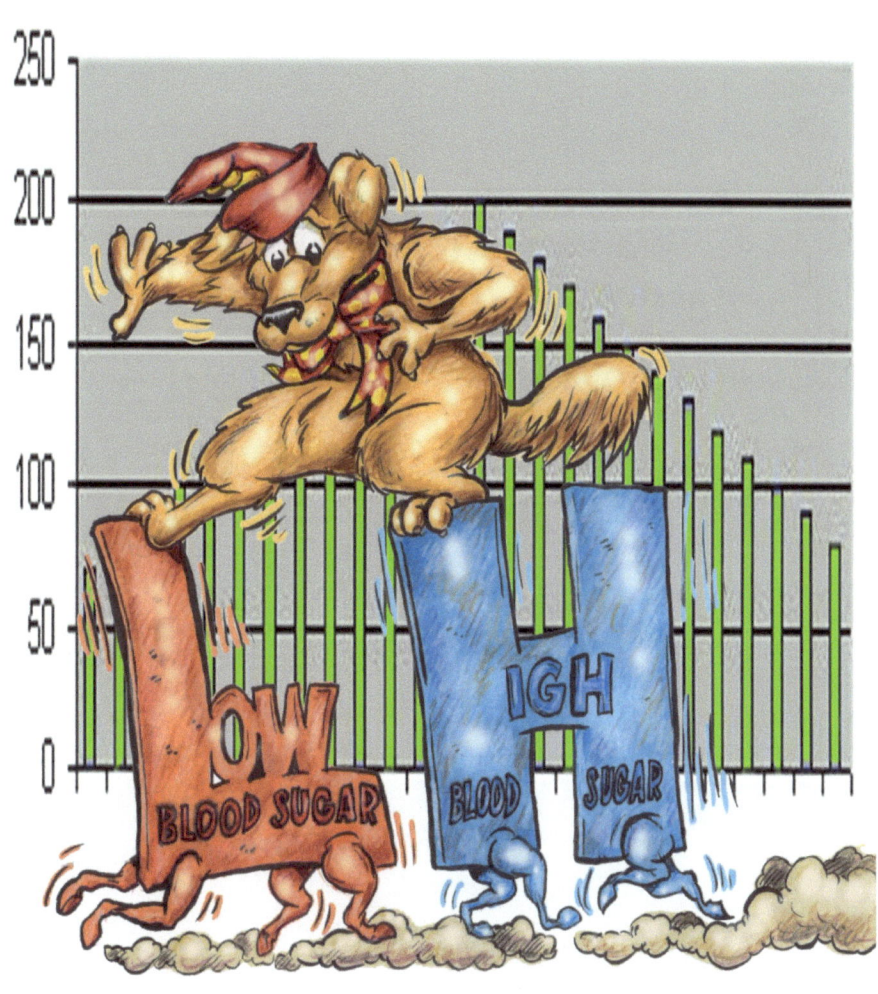

As long as Max and Winston
were able to do this
succesfully, life was good!

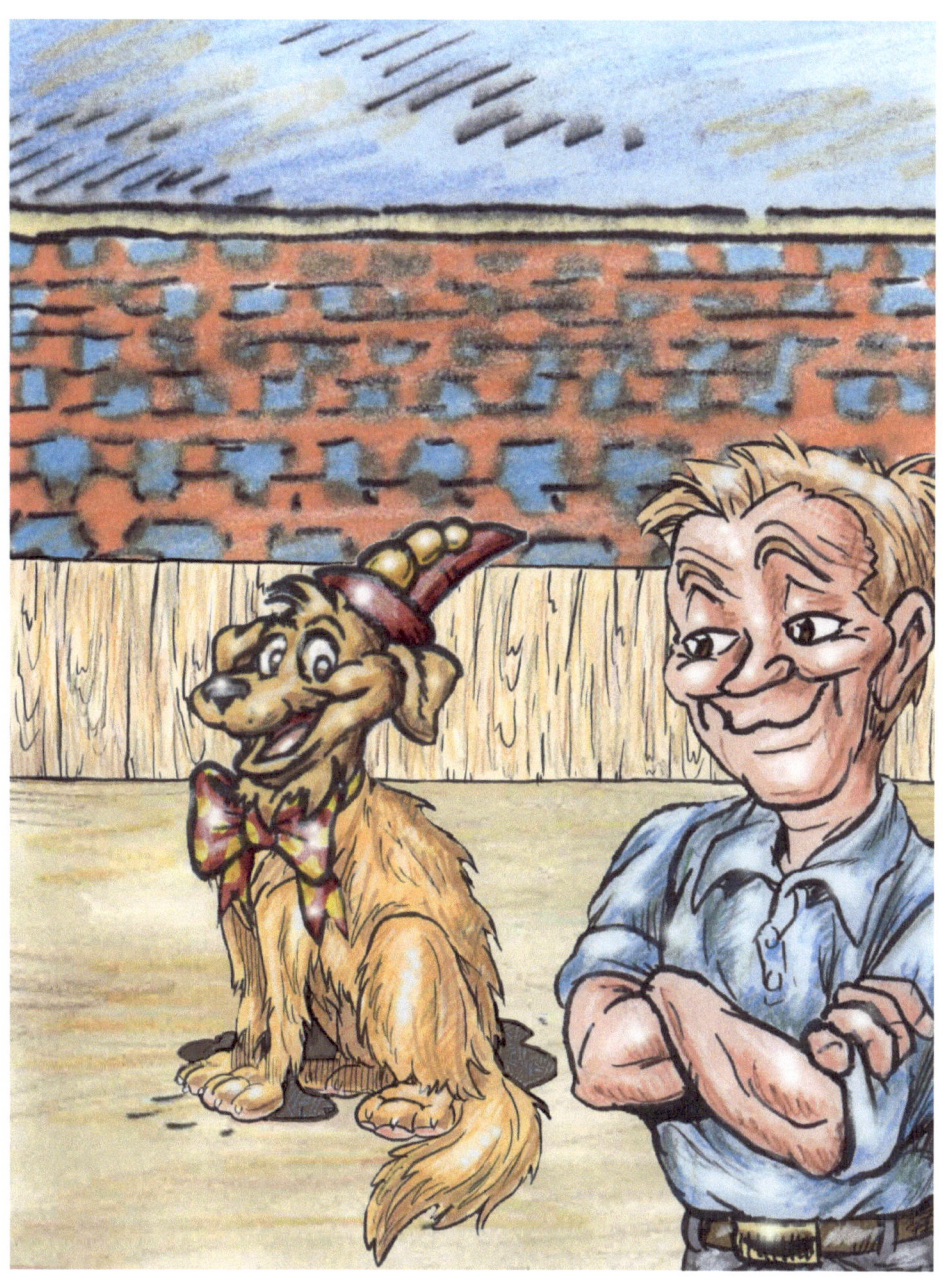

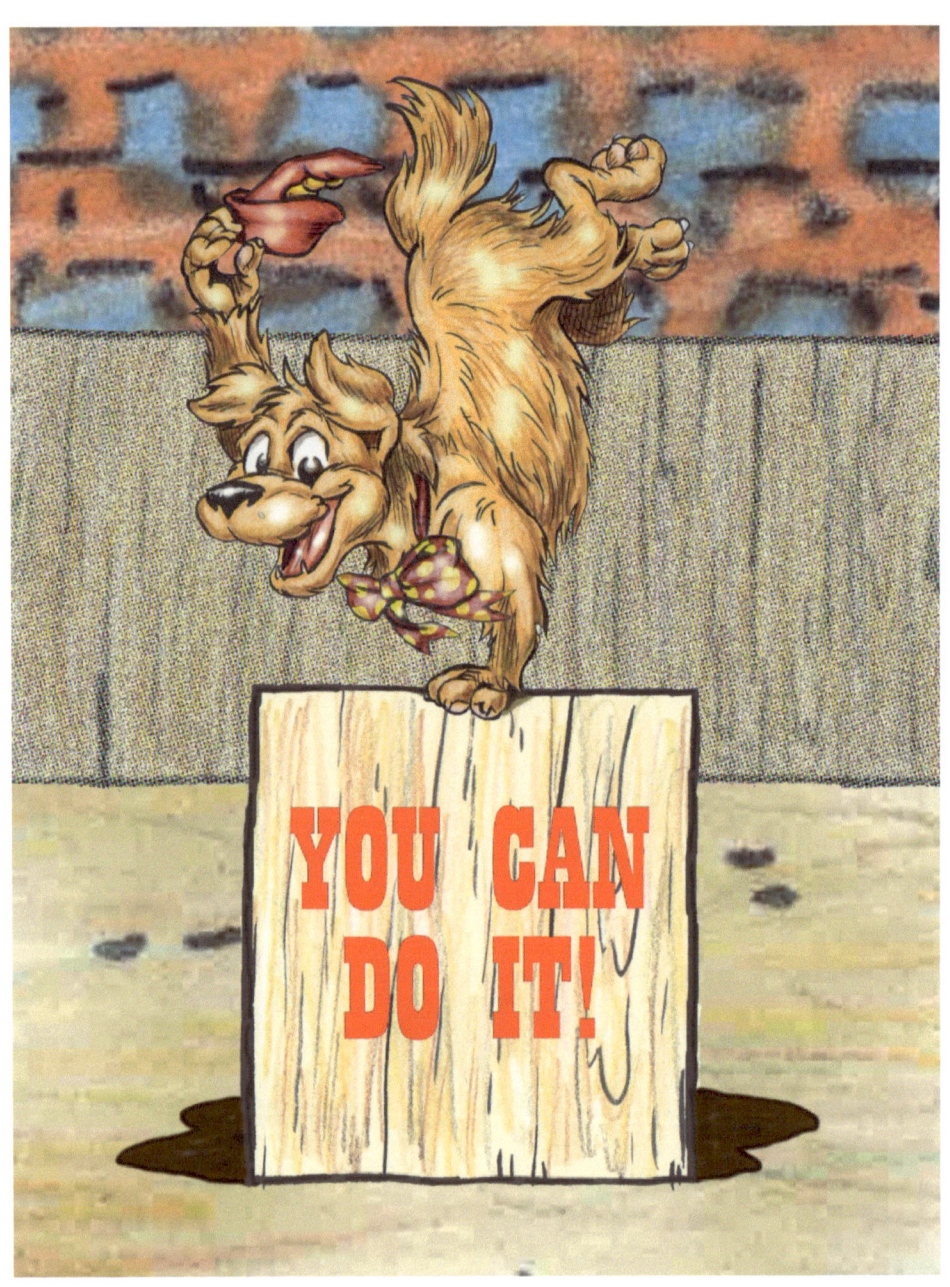

www.ingramcontent.com/pod-product-compliance
Lightning Source LLC
Chambersburg PA
CBHW041525280526
45792CB00004B/1388